Cosmetic Cupping

A Detailed Guide on the Use of Cupping for Beauty and Weight Loss

MARY CONRAD

ISBN: 1977582338
ISBN-13: 978-1977582331

DEDICATION

This is for my husband who is sitting on the desk watching stuff on YouTube. Lol. Thank you for your patience with me writing most of the time. !

MARY CONRAD

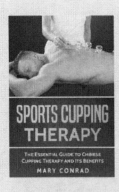

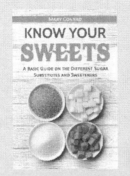

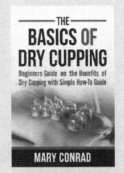

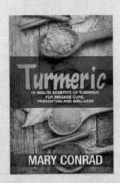

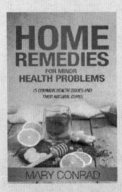

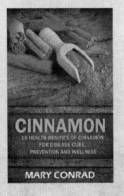

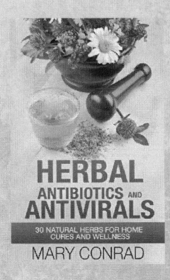

Disclaimer

This book provides general information, personal experiences and extensive research regarding health and related subjects. The information provided in this book, and in any linked materials, is based on my own personal experience and is for informational purposes only. It is not intended to be interpreted as a professional medical advice. Speak with your physician or a trusted healthcare professional prior to taking any nutritional or herbal supplements. Please keep in mind that reactions and results may vary from each individual due to differences in state of health

Before considering any guidance from this book, please ensure you do not have any underlying health conditions, which may interfere with the suggested healing methods. If the reader or any other person has a medical concern or pre-existing condition, please consult with an appropriately licensed physician or healthcare professional. Never disregard professional medical advice or delay in seeking it because of something you have read in this book or in any linked materials.

Table of Contents

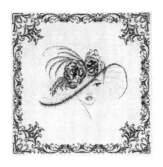

Introduction

Women go through different measures to achieve beauty goals. Some take the natural route while others choose to undergo the knife. Neither options are easy or painless. The natural route has one benefit though. For the most part, you don't have to worry about taking care of a post- operative wound healing or looking puffy, red and inflamed after an operation.

Cosmetic cupping is gaining popularity as a beauty regimen. The main reason is because it's easy to do. If you have the right type of cups at home and some oil you're pretty much good do go! Another benefit is that you don't need any deep knowledge on the cupping points, acupuncture points and the muscle physiology. The most that you'll need to remember would be to avoid large veins and arteries. This cupping technique helps with toning the skin, lessening the appearance of cellulite and assists in weight loss.

This book will look into the different uses of cupping for cosmetic purposes. It will include the basic techniques on how to perform cupping for toning, cellulite and weight loss. I'll also discuss the contraindications of the treatment, when to perform the treatment and what to expect.

The procedure is not rocket science but there are a few reminders that might help in getting better results from your treatment. Just a reminder is that this is not a miracle cure for cellulite, nor does it make you lose 30 pounds in one month. This procedure can improve and assist with those problems but it isn't a cure-all. Like any other natural procedure, it invests in your time and saves you money. With that said, let's take the journey together and find out more about cosmetic cupping and how you can add it to your beauty regimen.

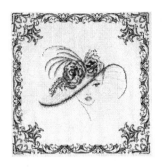

Chapter 1

What is Cosmetic Cupping

Cosmetic cupping is the use of cupping to improve the physical appearance of both the face and the body. It is usually performed with the use of silicone cups in key areas of the body such as the face, arms, thighs and stomach.

It is a new concept of applying the old methods of cupping for the beauty woes of today. Although I'm sure cellulite existed before this century, today's standards have become quite critical of any imperfection – natural or otherwise. Even with the worldwide call for a more realistic and natural beauty, some of us do want to lessen the appearance of cellulite or tone parts of our body for ourselves as part of being an empowered woman.

How does cosmetic cupping work?

Cosmetic cupping is the same as traditional cupping. It works by creating a negative pressure within the cup which creates a suction that pulls the skin outward. This in turn pulls the interstitial fluids from the tissues underneath the skin.

In the TCM (Traditional Chinese Medicine) perspective, it is believed that the suction draws the stagnant blood from the tissues towards the skin. The stagnant blood contains the toxins that have accumulated in the body. The result is a circular mark that looks similar to a bruise. The application of the cups activates the lymphatic system. This in turn helps facilitate the removal of the toxins from the body.

Cosmetic cupping primarily uses light flash/empty cupping together with massage cupping. It usually leaves minimal marks on the skin. If there are any, it'll disappear in a day or two. The focus of cosmetic cupping is to get the blood and energy flowing underneath skin. This helps in rejuvenating the skin.

Who can perform cosmetic cupping?

Anyone who is trained for cosmetic cupping can do the treatment. This can be seen offered in spas and clinics. Traditional cupping therapists can also perform cosmetic cupping. They have the added benefit of a thorough assessment of your current health status prior to the procedure.

When can cosmetic cupping be used?

As I've stated earlier, cosmetic cupping is usually used for three main purposes:

- To tone different areas of the body
- To reduce the appearance of cellulite
- Used in conjunction with a weight loss program

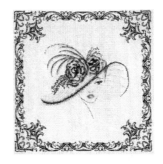

Chapter 2

Before the Procedure

There are a few reminders before undergoing this treatment. This chapter will discuss the contraindications, precautions, and what to expect.

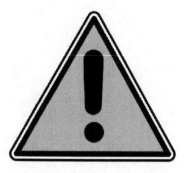

Precautions and Contraindications

Before trying this procedure, you need to consider your overall health as well as any known allergies to specific oils. If you have any chronic conditions such as autoimmune diseases or skin conditions, consult your healthcare provider prior to getting the service.

- If you have any open wounds, cupping should not be performed since it might cause the wound to bleed. This will place you at risk for an infection. The same goes for any trauma or bruises.

- If you have any inflammation or injury in the treatment site, cupping should not be performed since it can aggravate the inflammation and only cause more discomfort.

- If the client is dehydrated, cupping is contraindicated. Advise the client to rehydrate prior to the procedure.

- Precaution needs to be taken if the client is taking any anti-coagulants and blood thinners.

- Cupping should not be performed on the eyes, genitals, those who had cardiac arrest in the last 6 months and after the sixth month of pregnancy.

- It's contraindicated for all forms of acute and infectious diseases.

Preparation Prior to Cosmetic Cupping

Warm the area using a with a towel. There are different ways to do this. You can either use a towel warmer or place the towel over a bowl of hot water. Apply the towel on the treatment area and gently massage it. This preparation doesn't apply to facial cupping.

Prepare the correct cup size, which can depend on where you plan to have the procedure done. Smaller sizes are used for facial cupping. The common cup type is a cup with a suction bulb at the top, another option is using silicone cups, which comes in various sizes.

Plan where the cups will be placed. The direction of the cups for massage cupping will always be towards the lymph nodes. Also, large arteries and veins should also be avoided since it can divert the blood flow.

Note: For the treatment provider, they can provide information on the benefits of the procedure, the contraindication and have the client sign a consent form for the treatment.

What to expect during the treatment

The intensity of the cupping for cosmetic purposes is usually light cupping. It shouldn't be painful but there will be a "pulling" sensation. If there's any serious discomfort or pain, inform the treatment provider so they can adjust the intensity or stop the procedure.

For the initial treatment, the cups aren't usually left on the skin for more than 2 minutes. Doing this will leave visible marks which might not be flattering especially when it's on the face. The treatment provider will start with the least intensity and the minimum time frame for the treatment. This is to allow your skin to get used to the suction gradually. For the following sessions, the time may be lengthened.

Cosmetic cupping is a combination of flash cupping and massage cupping. Both may be used as the interchangeably depending on the initial assessment of your skin or for the specific purpose it's being used.

Terms

Effleurage – is a massage technique that uses the palm of the hand. The hand is moved in circular motion over the area.

Petrissage – is a massage technique that involves kneading the body.

Empty or Flash Cupping – cups are placed on the skin for a few seconds and then removed right away. This technique is usually done several times throughout the time of treatment. It's mainly used to stimulate the Qi without causing weakness after the treatment or leaving marks.

Massage Cupping – this cupping technique involves moving the cups while holding the suction. This is done by placing the cups on the skin, creating a vacuum using a pump gun or suction valve.

Light Cupping - this uses gentle suction. The skin is only slightly raised within the cup

Medium Cupping – this uses firm suction. The skin is moderately raised within the cup. The suction often feels "just right". The "pulling" sensation is felt more using this intensity.

Strong Cupping – this uses a strong suction that pulls on a lot of skin. The skin inside the cup will appear dark red and blotchy when using this technique. It can't be used for long periods of time in situ since it can cause discomfort.

MARY CONRAD

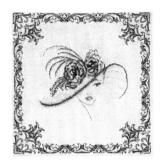

Chapter 3

Massage Cupping

Massage cupping will be used liberally throughout the process of cosmetic cupping. This chapter will tackle the basics.

Massage cupping is also called moving cupping. As stated previously, it involves moving the cup over a certain area while making sure the suction is in the cup.

There is a big difference when massage cupping is done by a TCM practitioner. These practitioners usually use this to address a problem in the body. Strong cupping is used which makes the procedure very uncomfortable and probably painful. However, it's one of the methods employed by athletes for post-training recovery. When done for cosmetic purposes, it's usually done with light to medium cupping depending on individual tolerance for the treatment and sensation.

Benefits:

✓ Massage cupping helps get the body fluids moving. This in turn assists in increasing the function of the lymphatic system. This system is responsible in excreting toxins from the body.

✓ It's relaxing. It loosens the fascia, which allows for smoother movement.

Preparation:

- Single cup (this can be silicone, rubber or glass)
- Oil

How-to:

1. Position the patient in a way that's convenient for the procedure.
2. Liberally apply the oil on the skin in long strokes (effleurage).
3. Place the cup on the treatment site and create a light suction.
4. Move the cup towards the direction of the lymph nodes. When moving the cup, use one hand to support (hold and manipulate) the movement of the cup while the other hand is pressed onto the skin for a smoother glide.
5. Observe the marks. It should be pink and bright and light enough to disappear within a day or two.

LYMPHATIC SYSTEM

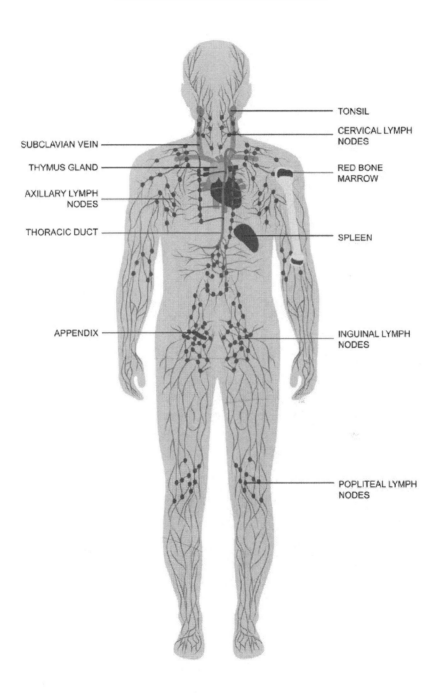

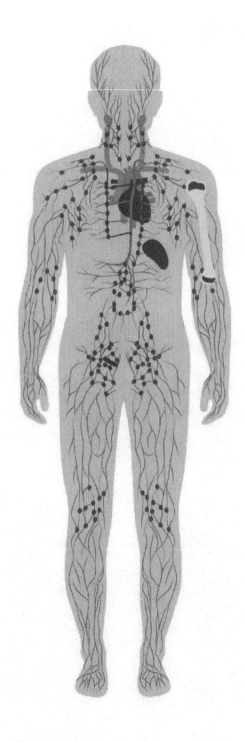

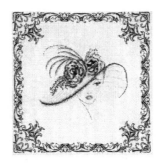

Chapter 4

Cosmetic Cupping for Toning

The proceeding chapters will look into the different ways that cosmetic cupping can be used. It'll also discuss the methods on how-to perform general procedures in different body parts that people commonly have issues with.

Cupping for Toning

According to TCM practitioners, cupping has the ability to increase the local metabolic patterns. The increase in local metabolic patterns is attributed to the increase in blood supply as well as lymphatic activity. The combination of increased blood flow, toxin removal and increased local metabolism results in toning.

How-to:

1. Apply oil liberally on the target area for treatment.
2. Warm the area using a warm towel or by gentle hand massage. You can do effleurage and petrissage on the area.
3. Perform moving cupping on the treatment site.
4. Continue for 5-10 minutes until the area is bright pink. This can differ per client. If they experience any sensitivity on the area, stop the procedure and let the skin rest. Move to another area.

Tip: Follow the contour of the body for an easier glide.

There are different parts of the body that can be cupped. Each one has a few minor differences that will be mentioned in the different sections below:

Cupping the Neck

The neck is sensitive to pressure and has thin skin with arteries and veins in certain areas. Cupping it is possible but always employ a light cupping intensity and avoid leaving the cup in situ.

1. Use one cup, preferably silicone. Oil the area.
2. Start with a light suction above the clavicle moving upward towards the chin or on either side of the neck.
3. You can repeat the second step, five to seven times.
4. Stop if there are any serious discomfort felt.

Cupping the Chest

When cupping this area, it will only involve the sternum and the upper chest (right below the clavicle). It will not pass by any other part.

Using a pump gun vacuum cupping set or a silicone cup, create a light or medium intensity suction on the middle of the sternum. Move the cup upwards towards the clavicle. You can repeat this several times until the skin is pink.

Cupping the Arm

Palpate where the clavicle ends, apply medium cupping on the area. Move the cup towards the biceps then triceps until just above the elbow. Please note that there are a set of nerves in the area that might get hit, so take a bit of precaution when doing this. The duration can be between 5 to 10 minutes.

Cupping the Abdomen

The abdomen holds a lot of the organs in the body, which is usually layered with some fat. When doing cupping for this area, light cupping, flash cupping and moving cupping can be performed.

When cupping the abdomen, the client should neither be hungry or full. Ideally, they need to be somewhere in between. An hour and a half to two hours after a meal is a good time to begin the cupping session.

1. Have the patient lie on his back.
2. Apply oil all over the treatment area.
3. For the first 10 minutes, apply random cups all over the stomach until it covers most of the area.
4. Use flash or empty cupping for the first 10 minutes. After covering the area with cups, remove it right away then reapply it.
5. After the 10 minutes are done, proceed with light moving or massage cupping. The duration will be for another 10 minutes.
6. Start at the sternum then move the cups outward.
7. When cupping the area near the umbilicus, you need to cup

around it clockwise moving the cup outward as you go.

8. The treatment time can be increased with successive visits up to 50 minutes.

Cupping the Thigh

In cupping the thighs, light, medium and strong cupping can be used. The intensity will again depend on the tolerance of the client. The muscles along the inner thigh can be more sensitive than the rest, so it might be prudent to take note of that prior to the treatment.

For massage cupping in the area, use a single cup. Apply oil on the treatment area. Place the cups on the site. Move it according to the muscle contour. Continue the treatment between 5-10 minutes for the initial treatment.

Cupping the Legs

The back of the legs can be sensitive so the best cupping intensity is between light and medium cupping. Start right below the knee and move the cup towards the feet. If the suction is maintained, you can rotate the cup back towards the knee. It has the same initial time frame as the rest.

Cupping the Buttocks

This is a great way to tone the area.

1. Use a single silicone cup. Oil the area liberally.
2. Medium cupping can be done comfortably in this area. For successive sessions, the provider can use strong cupping if well tolerated by the client.
3. There are two strokes that can be performed on this area. Starting from the outer portion of the buttocks, move the cup

towards the upper thigh, then move the cups upward, straight through the gluteus maximus. Stop the stroke on the lower back.

4. The second stroke starts at the middle of the flank. The cup is moved across the buttock towards the hip joint in an outward motion.

5. Duration is at 5-10 minutes for the first treatment.

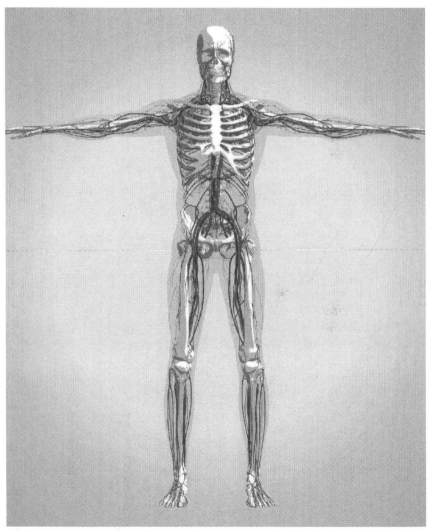

Fig. 1: Location of large vessels and bones in the body.

MARY CONRAD

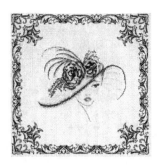

Chapter 5

Cupping for Cellulite Reduction

This is the most popular reason why people chose to try cupping. However, it is not a miracle cure for cellulite. It does minimize the appearance of it with frequent use, which is awesome since it only takes a few minutes daily and it can be done at home with some creativity and flexibility.

Cellulite according to Science

Cellulite is caused by a mixture of different factors. However, the definition of the condition is that it is the herniation of the subcutaneous fat from the connective tissue to the skin, which is evidenced by skin dimpling.

What Causes Cellulite:

Cellulite occurs in 80-90% of post-pubescent women. There are several factors attributed to help in the development of cellulite. It isn't quite clear how this forms exactly since it hasn't really been studied all that much. However, here is a list of the possible causes:

Hormones: The appearance of cellulite usually happens after puberty. There's no clinical evidence of which of the hormones are responsible but estrogen is suspected to be one of the major contributor to its formation. The main reason is that it happens with a lot of women but not with men.

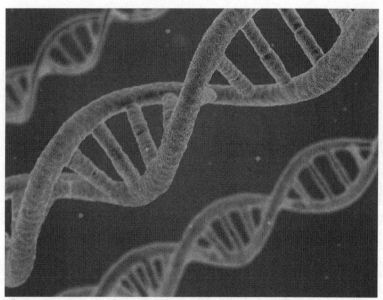

Genes: In a study done by Enzo Emmanuel, he used genetic study to determine links regarding the formation of cellulite. He discovered that specific genes and polymorphisms did have some link to the development of this cosmetic problem, specifically angiotensin converting enzyme (ACE) and hypoxia-inducible factor 1A (HIF1a) genes.

Non-modifiable factors: This includes factors such as race, body type, and the individual fat distribution.

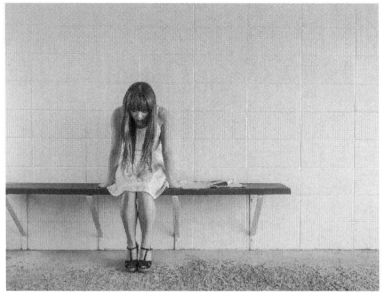

Lifestyle: Stress may contribute to the formation of cellulite. This is due to one chemical (catecholamines) that is released during times of stress.

How Cupping for Cellulite Reduction Works:

According to the TCM principle, cellulite is formed from poor lymphatic circulation which leads to lipid accumulation underneath the skin. Cupping addresses this issue by increasing the blood flow and getting the body fluids moving underneath the skin.

Reminders:

✓ Results can take up to 3 months before becoming noticeable. However, in conjunction with exercise (an hour of walking or running), it can be shortened.
✓ Drink the recommended amounts of water and make sure to be well hydrated.

How-to:

Since cellulite often occurs around the buttocks and upper leg. This section will provide information on how to cup those areas.

1. Position the patient according to the location of the cellulite. If it's on the back and front, start with the back.
2. Back: Oil the leg from the ankle up to the hip bones.
3. Front: Start oiling from the knee up to the groin area.
4. Warm the area using basic massage techniques (effleurage and petrissage).
5. For the initial treatment, use only light massage cupping and flash cupping. The duration is limited to 10 minutes. For the following sessions, you can increase the duration for 5-7 minutes with a maximum of 30 minutes for each treatment area.
6. Back: Once you have the cups in place, start either light massage cupping or flash cupping at the back of the lower leg (gastrocnemius). Work your way up towards the thighs and buttocks. Stop when you reach the iliac crest.
7. Front: Start at the knee area and work upwards. Note for the sensitive areas of the body.
8. As mentioned earlier, the direction of the treatment should be towards the location of the lymph nodes inside the body.

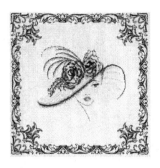

Chapter 6

Cupping in Conjunction with Weight Loss

In some parts of Asia, cupping is used together with a weight loss program. In a way, this makes sense in the TCM principle since cupping increases **local metabolism** and **tones the skin**, which may benefit those who want to lose fat around the arms, abdomen and buttocks without having to deal with excess skin. The increase in localized blood flow and lymphatic circulation would also help in fat metabolism.

Cupping on its own doesn't make anyone lose weight. It is only used as a supplemental treatment on top of a workout regimen that includes: physical activity, a diet plan and discipline to follow through.

This treatment involves the use of electroacupucture adhesive pads applied to a specific area. This device provides low to medium frequency stimulation for 30 minutes. This is believed to help the fat breakdown by stimulating the muscles. After, several cups are placed all over the area. The practitioner will perform Flash cupping with medium to strong intensity throughout the site for 15 minutes for the initial procedure. The intensity and duration may increase for the successive treatment. Moving cupping can also be applied for 10 minutes after for relaxation, and to facilitate the removal of toxins.

For this particular procedure, it is best to get a certified professional. They'll be able to provide the best treatment and plan it according to your current weight loss program.

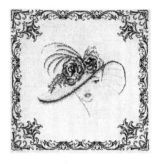

Chapter 7

Cupping the Face

Although it might sound a little intimidating, cupping the face is possible. However, the face has one of the thinnest skin throughout the body so it needs a gentle touch. Cupping the face brings the blood to the surface and increases blood circulation which brings both oxygen and nutrients to the area. This brightens the skin considerably.

According to the TCM principle, cupping may stimulate the skin to produce more collagen, which in turn results to firmer skin. The results can be visible by the sixth session.

Reminders:

- Facial cupping requires smaller cups for more gentle suction. It's more about stimulation. There should be little to no marks left on the skin after.

- There are various cups to choose from: silicone, rubber or a suction bulb Perspex cup. Any of these will do as long as it's the appropriate size. The sizes vary according to manufacturers.

- The color of the skin after cupping should be light pink and with no noticeable marks.

How-to:

1. Apply oil liberally throughout the face. You can apply anti-ageing oils or creams on the skin.
2. Massage the face with gentle sweeping movements from the chin moving upwards and outwards until the forehead.
3. Place the cup right at the center of the forehead move the cup upwards. Repeat the process as if smoothening out the creases between the eyebrows and the wrinkles on the center of the forehead.

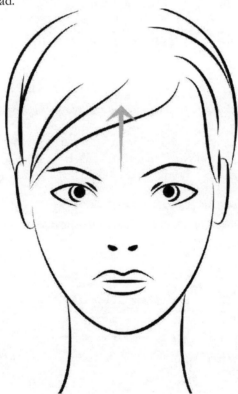

4. Move the cup on each side of the forehead right above the eyebrows.

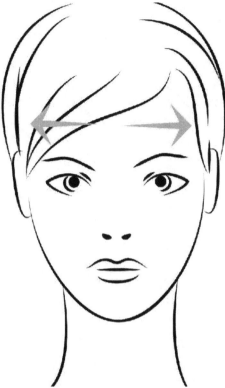

5. Place the cup underneath each eye and move it upwards and outwards.

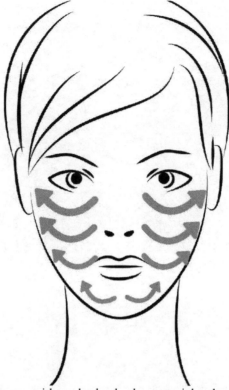

6. Do the same with each cheek, the area right above the mouth and the chin.
7. After, place the cup right at the temple. Create a light suction and move the cup downwards. The main reason for this is to direct the toxins towards the lymph nodes for excretion.

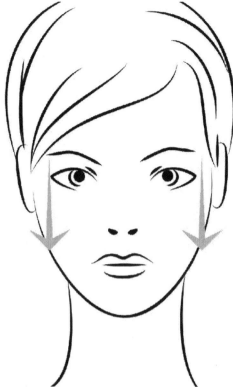

8. Continue moving cupping on the neck and underneath the collar bone (clavicle). For the scapula, move the cup outwards similar to the movements above. Continue the treatment for 10-15 minutes repeating the steps above.

MARY CONRAD

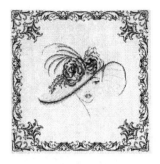

Chapter 8

Frequently Asked Questions

1. How long does each session last?

Initial session is always limited to 10 minutes, just to help the skin adjust to cupping. Sessions can be increased for 30-40 minutes or more depending on the treatment provider. It shouldn't last more than an hour.

2. How many times can I get treatment?

Once or twice weekly is the norm for Western version of cupping.

3. What do I do if I feel dizzy?

The movement of fluids and Qi can affect a small percentage of people causing dizziness. This is normal. Let the client sit down and have a drink of water or warm tea until the dizziness subsides.

4. Can I cup over skin moles?

No. Static cupping over moles is contraindicated.

5. When will I see a difference in my skin?

The difference may be visible within 6 sessions.

6. Can I bathe after a treatment?

Yes. However, make sure it is a warm bath.

7. Can I work-out or exercise or train after a session?

It isn't advised since it best to rest after a session. Cupping can be draining and exercise will expend more energy.

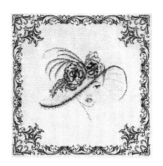

Conclusion

Cosmetic cupping is an intriguing new treatment that can be a game changer in your DIY beauty regimen. It has both benefits to your physical appearance as well as your health, which can't be said for most of the beauty trends out in the market today.

Like other natural products, cupping requires a certain amount of patience for results to be felt. It doesn't take one session of doing this at home or through a clinic or spa to see a difference but at least 6 sessions that can span for two weeks to a month depending on how often you want to have the session in a week.

I'm hoping that this book provided information and value on the basics of cosmetic cupping and how to perform it.

Finally, if you enjoyed this book, then I'd like to ask you for a favor. Would you be kind enough to leave a review for this book on Amazon? It'd be greatly appreciated!

Follow me on Facebook (Mary Conrad) and Twitter (@authormconrad).

Subscribe to my newsletter to get updates on my latest book and free giveaways!
www.maryconradrn.com

If you have any suggestions or specific natural remedies that you want to have researched and written, shoot me an email at authormaryconrad@gmail.com. I'm always on the lookout for great new topics to write about. :)

Have a great day!

Thank you for taking this journey with me, and good luck!

Author Biography

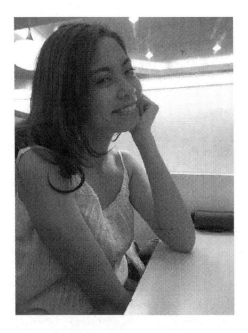

Mary Conrad is a Registered Nurse, who has a strong interest in natural remedies. As a mother, she believes in a holistic approach to health and well-being. Even though she graduated in the health profession, which usually advocates pharmaceutical medication, she believes that prevention is the best step towards health. Backed with scientific research, she wrote these books for both personal information and for others who share the same passion for holistic wellness. It's all about knowing the best natural ways to prevent disease and remedy current health problems. Like every health care provider, she believes in doing no harm, and promoting health. Take a step towards health, and towards nature.

CHECK OUT MY OTHER BOOKS:

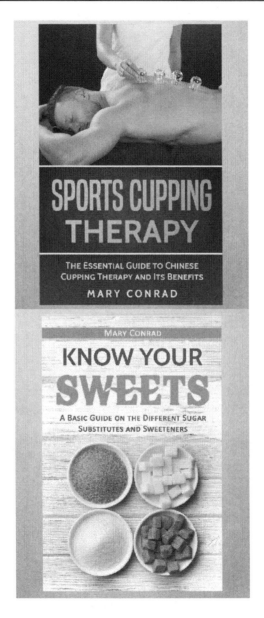

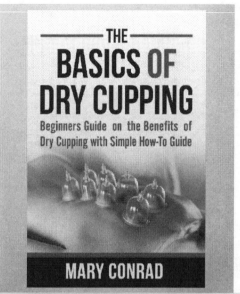

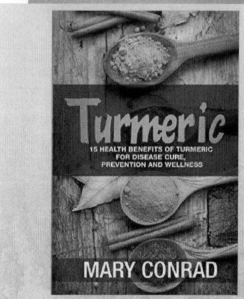

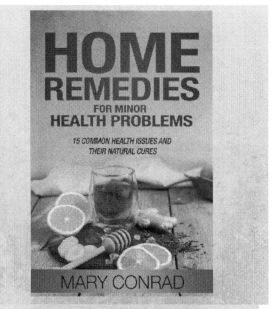

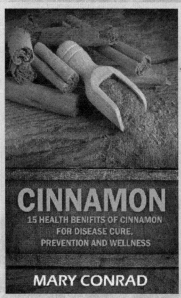

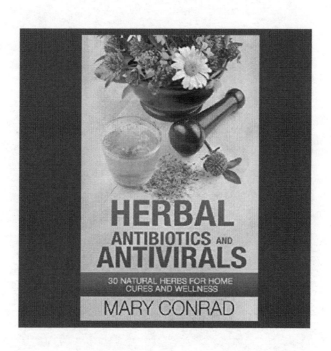

Made in the USA
Columbia, SC
27 November 2017